Pray.

Run.

A Food, Faith, and Fitness Guide
for
New and Renewed Runners

FOREWORD BY ERIC THOMAS, PH.D.

DAVID TROFORT

Eat. Pray. Run.
A Food, Faith, and Fitness Guide for New and Renewed Runners

By David Trofort

Icons by Juicy Fish, Freepik, Pixel Perfect, Kerismaker, Uniconlabs, and Edt.im.

Printed in the United States of America

ISBN 979-8-218-28351-3

Cover photo by iStock.com/Marco VDM

To contact the author:
DavidTrofort.com
eatprayrunbook.com

Dedication

To my wife Terra
and Nikolas, Myles, and Aaron, my amazing boys
I love you so much.

Contents

Foreword

From the moment I met my college friend and brother David, his passion for holistic well-being was evident. He possessed an innate understanding of the interconnectedness between our physical health, mental well-being, and spiritual growth. It was through our shared experiences in college ministry that I witnessed his unwavering commitment to empowering others to live a life of balance, purpose, and vitality.

In this book, David seamlessly weaves together his knowledge and experiences, offering readers a unique perspective on the synergy between nutrition, fitness, and faith. His extensive personal research and practical insights provide a comprehensive guide for individuals seeking to embrace a healthy lifestyle that encompasses all aspects of their being.

What sets David's approach apart is his unwavering belief that true wellness is a journey that transcends the physical. He delves into the importance of cultivating a positive mindset, nurturing healthy relationships, and seeking spiritual fulfillment. By combining scientific knowledge with a profound understanding of the human spirit, David invites readers to embark on a transformative journey that encompasses the body, mind, and soul.

Throughout the book, David's genuine care for his readers' health shines through. He effortlessly imparts his wisdom and expertise with an approachable and relatable tone, ensuring that everyone, regardless of their background or prior knowledge, can benefit from his insights.

Furthermore, David openly discusses the challenges *he* encountered on his own journey, emphasizing that the pursuit of wellness is not without its obstacles. Yet, he imparts invaluable lessons and offers a roadmap for overcoming adversity.

David's holistic slant to wellness is firmly grounded in his faith. He adeptly intertwines the principles of spirituality with practical guidance, demonstrating how nourishing our bodies and souls can go hand in hand. His insights indicate that well-being is not simply about achieving physical perfection, but about aligning ourselves with a higher purpose.

As I reflect on our time together in college ministry, I am reminded of the countless lives that David has positively impacted through music and the health ministry. His influence has inspired many to embrace a healthier lifestyle and embark on a transformative journey of their own. Welcome *Eat. Pray. Run.* as a valuable resource for *your* personal journey toward wellness, too.

~ Eric Thomas, **Ph.D.**

Introduction

The Power of *Eat. Pray. Run.*

What if you could improve your health and overall well-being by focusing on three, simple, logical things: eating well, cultivating a spiritual practice, and staying active?

That's the concept behind *Eat. Pray. Run.*, a holistic approach to comprehensive health and wellness that combines the power of food, faith, and fitness.

In today's fast-paced world, it's easy to overlook the value of these three areas of life. We may need more time to cook healthy meals or find time for prayer and meditation. Perhaps we need motivation to exercise regularly. Maybe available options are too overwhelming.

But here's the truth: If we prioritize food, faith, and fitness, we *can* improve our physical health, mental well-being, and overall quality of life.

How This Book is Organized

Part One of this book will explore nutrition's power and role in health. We'll discuss the benefits of a healthy diet and provide practical tips and strategies for meal planning, grocery shopping, and cooking healthy meals. We'll also look at mindful eating and how it can help us to make wiser, healthier food choices.

In Part Two, we'll shift to faith and spirituality, their mutual connection to health, and the many benefits of cultivating a spiritual habit. We'll discuss the power of prayer and meditation, along with useful tips for incorporating these practices into our daily lives. We'll also study how community and connecting with others can support our spiritual growth and health.

Part Three will focus on fitness and exercise. We'll delve into the many benefits of regular physical activity and will learn easy-to-apply tips for getting started with running. We'll also discuss why staying motivated is important and will share strategies for overcoming common obstacles to keeping active.

Finally, to help you see just how doable our holistic approach is, we'll share a few inspiring stories from those who have transformed their lives through *Eat. Pray. Run.*, including me.

Throughout the book, look for the following icons for easier reading and usage:

Eating-related information

 Faith and spirituality information

 Running/fitness information

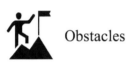 Obstacles

 Love information

 Benefits

 Testimonial

 Tips

Whether you're a new or renewed (meaning, starting over) runner, a devout believer, a spiritual seeker, or simply looking to improve your health and well-being, keep reading. By harnessing the power of food, faith, and fitness, you *can* become your best self.

Importance of Food, Faith, and Fitness

Food, faith, and fitness are all essential components of a healthy lifestyle with each playing a unique role in promoting physical, mental, and spiritual well-being:

Food: Grab the right bite! A healthy diet is key to maintaining healthy body weight, reducing the risk of chronic diseases, such as heart disease and diabetes, and improving overall health and energy levels. Eating a diet rich in fruits, vegetables, whole grains, lean protein, and healthy fats gives the body the nutrients it needs to function properly. In addition, mindful eating practices, such as paying attention to hunger and fullness cues, can help you make healthier food choices and improve your relationship with food.

Faith and spirituality: Believe in something positive! Studies have shown that people with strong faith or spiritual practice tend to have lower rates of depression and anxiety, better coping skills, and greater overall life satisfaction. Prayer, meditation, and attending religious services can help manage stress, define your purpose in life, and connect you with a supportive community.

Regular physical activity: Get moving! Being active regularly is crucial for maintaining a healthy body weight, reducing the risk of chronic diseases, and improving mental health and well-being. Exercise helps to strengthen muscles and bones, boost energy levels, and improve cardiovascular health. And regular movement can help reduce symptoms related to anxiety and depression, and improve your mood and self-esteem.

So, let's get started together to learn more!

Chapter 1: The Power of Nutrition

A serious crisis is confronting health professionals worldwide: Despite advances in pharmacology and extensive human and financial efforts in the health sector, they can't adequately treat chronic, noncommunicable diseases (NCDs). And the odds are astounding:

- NCDs make up almost 70% of the 55 million annual deaths worldwide.

- More than 50% of all Disability Adjusted Life Years (DALY) describe the years lost due to poor health, disability, and early death.

But is diet the primary reason for people's exceptional health and longevity? Let's see as we begin Part One, the food or "eat" section of *Eat. Pray. Run.*

How What We Eat Affects Our Health

Nutrients, Food's Building Blocks

Nutrients consist of carbohydrates, proteins, fats, vitamins, minerals, and water. The science of nutrition studies how the body uses each of these components to maintain and improve optimal physical and mental health. A balanced, healthy diet that includes a variety of nutrient-dense foods from each of these categories is crucial for proper nutrition.

But all it takes is a vacation … wedding … lunch … dinner … meeting … date … break in your day … party … holiday … life … to make you fall off the eat-right wagon and drift away from your goals.

And *how* we control our appetite can affect our mood, attitude, behavior, health, and quality of life. Sometimes being on a diet or fast, or inconsistently eating clean or healthy, can bring out the monster in us.

Why? Because we all – *me* included – love to eat. Eating is king! And it's often the best part of our day, bringing joy and happiness to life. From comfort food to junk food, we all indulge, no matter who we are or where we're from.

But here's the problem: If we love to eat and don't blend in eating balanced meals, then there's a high probability we aren't healthy or won't experience our best selves.

▶ **Food Works as Building Material and Body Fuel**
Every single bodily function depends on an adequate supply of nutrients and the correct nutrient processing, meaning metabolism. Proteins, for example, serve as structural elements and components of enzymes, which are our metabolism's engines. Carbohydrates primarily provide energy-dependent processes, and fatty acids fulfill cell communication tasks, plus structure-forming and energy-supplying functions.

But our food provides much more than just energy. It also provides essential substances, such as vitamins and minerals, vital cofactors for our metabolism.

Considering all these aspects, it's clear that quantity and the composition of our food profoundly affect our development and bodily functions. Having not enough and/or too much of one or more nutrients can lead to issues, such as deficiency symptoms, premature aging, or NCDs.

How Diet Affects Genes

Food and its components are more than nutrients for our hardware and energy metabolism. Studies show that diet affects our genes, and it does so across generations. This effect is called epigenetics, or as the Centers for Disease Control and Prevention says, the study of how our behaviors and environment can cause changes that affect how our genes work.

The influence of diet is critical, including affecting the developing fetus, as well as potentially materializing later in the child's life as obesity, insulin resistance, type 2 diabetes, and eating preferences.

Although we obviously didn't shape our mothers' diet, we *can* influence our genes epigenetically with our diet. Various studies on humans, animals, and cell cultures have shown that both macro and micronutrients and phytochemicals from food, such as flavonoids, carotenoids, coumarins, and phytosterols, are directly involved in metabolic reactions and even regulate genes' functions.

Nutrition's Role With Chronic Diseases

There's a strong link between nutrition and the prevention of chronic diseases. While these diseases often occur due to genetic, lifestyle, and environmental factors, poor nutrition also is a leading cause. As a result, here's what can happen:

Disease Types	Deficient Diet Choices	Potential Risks
Cardiovascular	High in saturated & trans fats, cholesterol, sodium	High blood pressure, arterial plaque buildup, heart attack, stroke
Type 2 diabetes	High in sugar, refined carbs, unhealthy fats	Insulin resistance, obesity, fatigue, sluggishness
Cancer	High in processed & red meats, saturated & trans fats, sugar	Colon, breast, prostate cancers
Osteoporosis	Low in calcium, vitamin D	Weak, brittle bones
Brain	High in saturated & trans fats, low in antioxidants, omega-3 fatty acids	Cognitive decline, Alzheimer's, dementia

Nutrition and Mental Health

Besides *physical* health, the nutrients we consume also affect our *mental* health. Consider this:

Mental Health Symptoms	Better Diet Choices	Better Outcomes
Depression and anxiety	Whole foods, fruits, vegetables, healthy fats	Reduced symptoms of depression and anxiety
Moodiness and depression	Omega-3 fatty acids in fatty fish, flaxseeds, & chia seeds, plus vitamins B, including folate, B6 and B12	Better brain health, mood and decreased risk of depression
Sleep and stress issues	Tryptophan (from foods such as turkey, chicken, eggs, & nuts) and magnesium (leafy greens, nuts, whole grains)	Better sleep quality and lowered stress

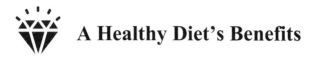 A Healthy Diet's Benefits

Here's what a balanced, properly portioned diet can do:

- **Reduce chronic-disease risks:** Add more fruits, vegetables, lean protein, healthy fats, and whole grains, such as brown rice and quinoa.

- **Reduce inflammation:** Add healthy fats, such as nuts, seeds, and fatty fish, to infuse antioxidants throughout your body and neutralize free radicals.

- **Gain less weight:** Eat fewer processed, refined foods to lower sugar, salt, and unhealthy fats intake.

- **Improve memory, attention, mood, and problem-solving skills:** Add more fruits, vegetables, whole grains, and omega-3 fatty acids.

- **Increase energy levels and sleep quality:** Add foods high in protein, healthy fats, and complex carbs.

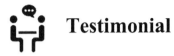 Testimonial

~ From author David Trofort

I realized eating's pitfalls many years ago. However, I didn't do much about it. My intense love for eating began during childhood. I was born in Brooklyn in 1971, and like most families, my parents André and Marie introduced me to food. I was the last of seven (the number of completion) amazing siblings: Margaret, Richard, Rachel, André Jr., Gabriel, and Eli.

Being the baby, I was quite spoiled and could do no wrong! And Margaret and Rachel were extremely protective of me, with Rachel claiming me as her very own.

But at mealtime, all that nurturing surrendered to a fend-for-yourself, survival-of-the-fittest competition! To ensure that I had more than scraps after my siblings' melee, my mother prepared my plate: "diri ak pwa" rice, red beans, and a piece of chicken, a staple in the traditional Haitian home. (The typical, alternative meal featured bologna or hotdogs.) And it was delightful!

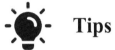 **Tips**

While medical studies indicate that diets with limited or no meat reduce the risk of heart disease and other ailments, remember: It's the overall quality of your *total* diet that influences your whole health. So, consider dining on:

- **Grilled chicken or fish** with a side of roasted vegetables
- **Stir-fry** with mixed vegetables and lean protein
- **A salad** with a variety of greens, vegetables, and a lean protein
- **An omelet** with vegetables and a slice of whole-grain toast

- **A plant-based diet**, omitting red meat for at least

  one meal

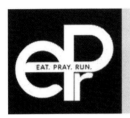

"Tell me what you eat,
and I will tell you what you are."

~ Jean Anthelme Brillat-Savarin

Chapter 2: Meal Planning

Meal planning is when you intentionally decide what you'll eat for a certain amount of time. But most of us – even when we know it's the right thing to do, even when we know nutrition is the key to lasting health – need more time and motivation to put meal planning into practice.

While it may be a bit daunting, there's no way around it: Meal planning and food prepping can help you stay on track with your healthy-eating goals. And cooking for yourself is the first step to addressing your health.

But before you do, remember that food interacts with your body's chemistry and gene makeup, including your epigenetics and body type *(see Chapter One)*. For example, while there are healthy vitamins, there also are natural pollutants on the organic shelf, and *your* body might react differently than someone else's to these items.

Regardless, meal planning is worth the effort. Here's how and why it can become a simpler, enjoyable part of your routine:

How to Create A Meal Plan

Define Plan's Duration

Set aside a day each week for planning what to eat over the next seven days. (A week is a good idea because it's short enough to preserve fresh food.) Use your favorite recipes to get started, or browse online to save recipes on your cell phone or read recipe books. Note that the total amount per grocery purchase is large, but not wasteful because you'll consume nearly everything.

Decide Your Medium

Select one of the following as your preferred way to map out your seven-day meal plan:

- A blackboard in your kitchen to write on with chalk

- A notebook

- A bullet planner

- A paper shopping list

- A clipbook

- An app (e.g., Plan to Eat or Eat This Much meal planner)

- A document you create on your laptop, cell phone, or tablet

Next, for each of the next seven days, fill out your meal plan, splitting up the days of the week with theme days. For example, you might want noodles on Tuesdays, rice on Wednesdays, potatoes on Thursdays, etc. If you wish to plan a week ahead, start planning the day after your grocery purchases.

Create Your "Idea" Store

Collect new and previously prepared recipes from online, cookbooks, magazines ... wherever you like. Then record the recipes you've chosen, using the medium you've selected. Next divide your recipes into categories, such as "Quick Dishes," "Cold Dishes," "Vegan Dishes," or "Asian Dishes," whatever suits you. Categories make it easier to create future meal plans.

Whichever process you choose, use it well to save as much time as possible.

Grocery Shopping

Your selected recipes will indicate what ingredients you'll shop for at the grocery store. Make sure to read food labels to make informed decisions, ensuring that the contents consist of whole foods without added sugars or artificial ingredients. Also look for foods with high amounts of nutrients per calorie.

Cooking Healthy Meals

So, you've planned and bought the right foods, but it's also equally important to cook everything properly.

For example, to retain food's nutrients, steam, bake, and roast your meals. Use herbs and spices, instead of salt, for flavor. Choose lean proteins, such as chicken, fish, and tofu, and limit your intake of red and processed meats. Incorporate a variety of colorful fruits and vegetables into your meals for a range of nutrients – not to mention, the incredible, boosted eye appeal of what's on your plate! And always experiment with healthy recipes and cooking techniques to keep meals interesting and enjoyable.

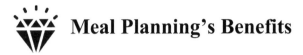 Meal Planning's Benefits

Healthiness

Deliberately plotting out and selecting which foods you'll eat usually means you'll:

- **Cook and freshly prepare** more balanced meals for yourself. That way, *you* control what's in your food.

- **Stay on track** with your healthy-eating goals.

- **Lessen the enticement** of making impulse purchases because you'll already have what you need at home.

- **Vary your diet more,** noting which foods you eat too often or neglect.

- **Lift your soul:** You no longer spend the whole day at work thinking about what to shop for and cook in the evening because you've already planned it.

Sustainability

When you meal plan, shop with an environmentally conscious mindset. Consequently, you'll:

- **Visit the grocery** store less often, using less gas to pollute the air than with no planning.

- **Eat more fresh produce,** reducing package waste versus purchasing ready-made, processed food encased in paper or plastic. (Skip in-store, pre-chopped, packaged produce. Instead, buy full sizes to cut and sort them yourself at home. They'll be handy for quick, easy snacking, and you'll likely satisfy the daily recommended amount, too.)

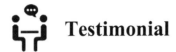 Testimonial

~ From Mark J.

My health journey, back in the day, was null and void. I wasn't watching what I would eat … I was taking blood pressure medicine, I got up close to about 400 pounds, headed in the wrong direction. In 2013 or 2014, it really hit me that I needed to do something about it.

I had weight-loss surgery in October 2014. In January 2015, I picked up running. I got on the treadmill, would start off and walk five minutes, and run a minute, then walk a minute, run a minute, for 30 minutes. The next week, I would run two minutes, walk a minute, three minutes, five minutes … that's how I built myself up.

Then I connected with [author David] and that friendly competition gave me motivation to keep going.

I started running half-marathons, 5Ks, 6Ks. I'm exercising about three or four days a week now … I try to eat what's healthy, a lot of vegetables, fruits and lean meats. I don't eat like I used to eat, just overindulge. Every now and then, I'll treat myself in moderation.

By being a believer, it gives me faith that I know that I can do this walk as I walk in Christ. I'm praying to God every day to give me strength in this journey … to get up and work out, even when I don't feel like it, and to give me the strength to eat right. It's a faith walk. *Eat. Pray. Run.* personally – and I know it's going to help the world – helped me. I wouldn't be at this place in my running journey if it wasn't for [David].

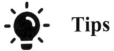 # Tips

To simplify meal planning and cooking, as well as make eating healthier and fun:

- **Set aside time each week** to plan out your meals and snacks for the upcoming week.

- **Make a list** *before* you visit the grocery store and adhere to it. This can help you avoid impulse buys and stick to your healthy-eating goals.

- **Shop the store's perimeter** to find fresh produce, lean proteins, and dairy products.

- **Look for sales** and coupons to save money on healthy foods.

- **Purchase frozen fruits and vegetables**. They're as nutritious as fresh produce and last longer.

- **Prepare meals beforehand** to save time during busy weekdays.

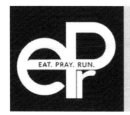

"For tomorrow belongs to the people who prepare for it today."

~ African proverb

Chapter 3: Mindful Eating

Mindfulness isn't new. It originally comes from Buddhism and has been practiced for 2,500 years. Then in 1979, renowned American molecular biologist Jon Kabat-Zinn, Ph.D., developed Mindfulness-Based Stress Reduction. He defined mindfulness as the "awareness that arises through paying attention, on purpose, in the present moment, nonjudgmentally."

However, Dr. Kabat-Zinn's philosophy and practice is counter to *our* society, which often focuses on achieving as much as possible and to always be "functioning." This constant demand for performance can easily lead to us ignoring our feelings, perceptions, and true needs in everyday life. And ultimately our habits and behavior take over, sometimes resulting in problematic eating.

But what if we take mindfulness – the art of *living* consciously (or turning off our autopilot) – and apply the same principles to mindful *eating*?

Here's how to begin the art of eating consciously:

How to Practice Mindful Eating

Mindful eating has nothing to do with a new diet, calorie counting, eating control, or excluding certain foods. Why? Because food is just food. Rather, mindful eating is about the *how* of eating or observing yourself while eating, perceiving without judging, no matter what and where we eat.

Quiz Yourself

To start mindful eating, ask these questions:

- When do I eat?

- Why am I eating?

- What is good for me when eating, and what nourishes me?

- How and where do I notice hunger?

- What does my food look like, what is its consistency, and how does it taste?

- How and where do I notice I'm full?

- What thoughts and emotions do I associate with eating?

- Where am I with my thoughts and feelings when I eat?

Assess Your Hunger

Before eating, take a moment to assess your level of hunger. While eating, pay attention to how full you feel, and stop eating when you are comfortably full.

Slow Down

Take time to chew your food thoroughly and savor each bite without watching TV or using your phone.

Be Present

Focus on your food's taste, texture, and smell. Take time to appreciate your food and the effort used to prepare it.

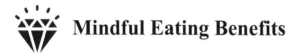 **Mindful Eating Benefits**

Improved Digestion

When we eat mindlessly, we either may chew improperly or eat too quickly, leading to indigestion and discomfort. Just slow down and pay attention to food to let the body digest and absorb nutrients fully and improve overall gut health.

Reduced Stress

Many people with obesity experience food-related guilt and regret due to widespread prejudice and stigmatization. Some also may react to loneliness or other unpleasant feelings, using food to hide their struggles. No matter the reasons, additional stress mounts, and sweets and snacks more frequently become "comfort" crutches.

However, if you adopt a benevolent and accepting attitude when eating mindfully, you can:

- Counteract feelings of guilt and, over time, develop a health-promoting relationship with food. (That's why mindfulness and mindful eating are important parts of eating-disorder therapies.)

- Be fully present at the moment without distractions, free to focus on your food's taste, texture, and smell.

- Discover and break negative behavioral patterns. By observing your thoughts, feelings, and perceptions before, during, and after eating, you can find your way back gradually to your actual needs.

Weight Management

When you hone in on hunger and fullness cues, you can recognize when you're full and stop eating. Otherwise, if you eat quickly, your stomach and brain may not respond with a feeling of fullness – or satiety – until after you've already consumed a large amount. This can leave you feeling overfull and sluggish.

Studies showing people who have learned mindfulness and practiced mindful eating found that they experienced fewer binge-eating episodes. Additionally, there's evidence that mindfulness practice can positively affect losing and maintaining weight *after* a diet.

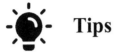 **Tips**

You've read these tips before because mindful eating is intimately connected to our previous two chapters. But it bears repeating:

- **Plan your meals** to avoid making hasty food choices and unhealthy snacking.

- **Choose healthy snacks** intentionally and those rich in nutrients.

- **Avoid mindless snacking**, especially when you're bored or stressed. Instead, focus on satisfying hunger.

- **Put down the fork**, taking breaks between small bites to feel fullness in between.

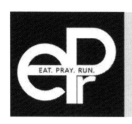

"Our life is shaped by our mind;
we become what we think."

~ Buddha

Chapter 4: Spirituality and Health

Now that we've completed the food or "eat" section, we're now beginning Part Two, the faith or "pray" portion of *Eat. Pray. Run.*

As with countless things in life, "spirituality" has a multitude of meanings. But Dr. Christina Puchalski, head of the George Washington Institute for Spirituality and Health, explains it as "each person's search for the meaning and ultimate purpose of life. This meaning can be found in religion, but it can often be broader than that, including the relationship with a divine figure or with transcendence, relationships with others."

In other words, spirituality is a personal belief system involving a higher power or force.

We often turn to faith, prayer, and meditation, all of which are aspects of spirituality, when we need to cope with stress, find meaning in our lives, and improve our mental and physical health. And for those seeking Christian theology's take on spirituality, we find the topic in at least 75 verses of the Bible, spanning seven books, including:

- "The Spirit of God has made me; and the breath of the Almighty gives me life." (Job 33:4)

- "Yet a time is coming and has now come when the true worshipers will worship the Father in spirit and truth, for they are the kind of worshipers the Father seeks. God is spirit, and his worshipers must worship in spirit and in truth." (John 4:23-24)

- "And if the Spirit of him who raised Jesus from the dead is living in you, he who raised Christ from the dead will also give life to your mortal bodies through his Spirit who lives in you." (Romans 8:11)

Let's look closer at how our quest for spirituality relates to our health:

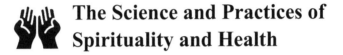 The Science and Practices of Spirituality and Health

The world suffers from constant chaos: COVID-19 and its after effects, earthquakes, hurricanes, tornadoes, floods, wars, famine, global warming, a haywire moral compass, and every kind of "ism" imaginable. While it seems like no entity is controlling this "ball of confusion," our omnipotent, omniscient God deliberately and creatively formed us to complete something quite special on this Earth.

And believe it or not, the best place to find that "something" to start is within.

What's the ideal way to "start within"? It's to meditate and pray, a centuries-old custom that today's physicians and researchers at America's elite universities still explore to determine the connection between spirituality and health.

Here's a broad, simple overview of what they've learned, plus insight into the community's influence on your spiritual growth:

Meditation

Meditation is when you stop and listen to your inner being. This involves focusing the mind on a particular object, thought, or activity to relax and attain mental clarity. Regular usage of this practice has been shown to reduce stress and anxiety, improve mood, enhance cognitive function, lower blood pressure, promote peace, and improve immune function.

Two popular meditation types are:

▶ **Transcendental meditation,** or when you use a specific mantra or sound for about 20 minutes, twice a day, to help quiet the mind and achieve deep relaxation.

▶ **Mindfulness** (as detailed in Chapter Three), when you pay attention to the present moment without judgment or distraction. You can practice mindfulness *anywhere* through deep breathing, body scanning (or focusing on your body in segments, starting at your feet and gradually working toward your head), and mindful eating.

Prayer

Prayer is food for the soul. It's a vital form of communication and spiritual development, presenting yourself directly to God. In its highest form, prayer is the pure expression of loving devotion to God. And, as with meditation, you can practice it within a religious or spiritual context or as a secular practice.

One type of prayer is prayers of the heart. These involve cultivating love, gratitude, and compassion toward yourself and others. We often associate this practice with religious traditions.

While many attest to prayer's power, others object to it because:

► **They don't believe:** No belief or a different concept of spirituality makes prayer feel meaningless or ineffective.

► **It triggers negativity:** Some have suffered guilt, shame, or fear to due religious-related or personal traumas.

► **They don't understand:** Prayer seems illogical because of the lack of exposure or proper education about the practice's purpose and benefits.

▶ **They're too busy:** Life is a whirlwind with overwhelming responsibilities, and there's not enough time or energy to add yet another task.

▶ **It just doesn't click:** Prayer doesn't resonate with everyone's personal preferences or values.

To pray or not to pray: It's everyone's choice because we have free will.

Yoga

Yoga is a physical and spiritual practice that began in ancient India. It combines physical postures, breathing techniques, and meditation to promote physical and mental well-being. As with meditation and mindfulness, yoga can reduce stress and anxiety, improve flexibility and balance, and enhance immune function.

Community Connection

As you integrate various "look within" techniques into your faith walk, it's essential to also include how finding community supports spiritual growth and health.

When the community provides a safe, empathetic environment, you're untethered to survey your beliefs, ask questions, and receive guidance and support among others who share similar values and experiences. This freedom works wonders, lessening feelings of isolation and strengthening a sense of belonging and acceptance, especially if family and friends aren't available or supportive.

Many spiritual communities offer classes, workshops, and retreats to help deepen your understanding of faith, self, and purpose. These opportunities can be uniquely valuable for spiritual newcomers or seasoned saints, variety seekers, or those experiencing existential crises.

And, for many, hearing perspectives and receiving mentoring from spiritual professionals and peers in communal settings serve as tremendous encouragement and accountability. And such counsel helps you to stay the course, reaching toward spiritual goals and commitments.

Of course, when you turn to your community for help, *you* can always serve others along the way. No spiritual gift or talent is too small or unneeded. And you're likely to *receive* more because you gave.

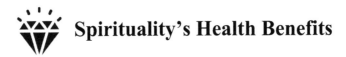 Spirituality's Health Benefits

Better Coping Mechanisms

Live long enough and something eventually will come along to challenge you. When it does, spirituality can help you cope better, providing comfort and support, especially when you exercise spiritual practices that address your meaning and purpose.

Enhanced Immunity

When something compromises your health, it's easy to feel like life is out of control or lacking logic. However, some have discovered that engaging with spiritual practices and beliefs can stimulate a sense of purpose and direction, boosting your ability to fight back and increase your overall emotional well-being.

Higher Connection

Via prayer, you can receive comfort, guidance, purpose, and help when feeling connected to something – a higher power or divine force – greater than you. Many also benefit from spiritual growth.

Improved Mental Health

Prayer can be a source of strength and support if you struggle with anxiety, depression, addiction, or other mental health challenges. For many, it provides hope, stamina, and mental clarity when navigating difficult experiences.

Improved Physical Health

Various studies cite that participating in spiritual and religious activities can help you live longer, enhance your immune function, and be sick less often. This may be due, in part, to spirituality reducing stress, a negative influence on the immune system.

Increased Resilience

Research has shown that the more spiritual or religious you are, the faster you could recover from a stroke and other chronic conditions. You also could acquire better coping skills and be more resilient in stressful situations.

More Gratitude

Prayer can nurture a sense of gratitude, shifting focus away from negative thoughts and toward a more positive outlook on life.

More Peace

If a situation arises requiring ongoing, intense management, spirituality can help you find peace and acceptance. This calmness can allow you to focus and cope better with the challenge and find ways to live a fulfilling life, despite the limitations.

Reduced Stress

Participating in spiritual practices, such as prayer, meditation, or attending religious services can have a calming, centering, grounding effect on the mind and body.

Prayer also can reduce your breathing, while promoting

concentration and lowering blood pressure.

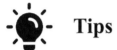 **Tips**

Here's how to incorporate spirituality into your daily life:

- **Find a quiet space**, be it indoors or outside, where you feel comfortable and are distraction free.

- **Set aside a specific time** each day to get quiet or centered. Consistency is key in establishing a daily practice.

- **Choose a mantra** or prayer that's meaningful to you, repeating it slowly and intentionally.

- **Start with short sessions,** a few minutes each day, and gradually increase your time.

- **Be patient.** If your mind wanders, and it probably will:

  - Acknowledge and release your thoughts, visualizing them as floating clouds or leaves.

  - Focus on a single point, such as a candle's flame or a religious figure or symbol, to gently redirect your mind to your mantra or prayer, and your breathing.

  - Use guided meditations, prayer books, videos, or classes.

  - Just keep going, even if you miss a day, and with no judgment.

- **Attend religious services** or gatherings regularly, connecting with like-minded people.

- **Seek guidance** from a teacher or mentor as you develop your practice.

- **Practice gratitude.** Reflect on what makes you grateful. It's hard to focus on negativity when you lock in on positivity.

- **Be kind.** Volunteer or help someone in need.

- **Connect with nature.** Walking outdoors or hiking can help you bond more with God's magnificently made, detailed elements and help you realize that *you* are still His most-loved and highest-prized creation.

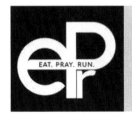

"At any moment, you have a choice, that either leads you closer to your spirit or further away from it."

~ Thich Nhat Hanh

Chapter 5: Fitness and Health

Within the previous eat and pray sections, we learned how food and faith interlink with our health. Fitness, meaning our physical and mental well-being for everyday efficiency, also rightly commands our attention to make our bodies their best.

Sure, *nearly everyone justifies not exercising* due to demanding responsibilities, no time or fitness equipment, gym membership costs, … you name it! But, like healthy eating, fitness is an essential part of an optimized lifestyle for a better quality of life.

Running is a workout for the whole body. The control center of movement, such as step length and frequency, transmits impulses to all moving parts, starting from the body's middle. This requires a healthy, muscular, basic tension in the mid-section, while the remaining muscles work to prevent sluggishness. Good body tension (a by-product of regular-strength training) also protects against excessive and incorrect strain when running.

Here's what else we can learn as we start – or restart – a well-thought-out training plan to get our *run* on:

How to Start Running

Consistently exercising for just 30 minutes a day, five times weekly, does a body good – from boosting your cardiovascular system to strengthening muscles to improving metabolism.

Experts now report that those 30 minutes *don't* have to occur in one session, but rather in shorter intervals! And practically any movement, like climbing stairs, vacuuming, carrying groceries, walking to your mailbox, etc., counts as exercise.

If you're a beginner and your training of choice is running, keep reading:

Get the Right Gear

Invest in good running, properly fitted, supportive shoes. Also, wear comfortable and moisture-wicking clothes that don't restrict your body movement.

Choose the Right Running Surface

The right running surface depends on the type of training you're doing, your risk and comfort tolerance, and your desired outcome. However, varying your run using all of the following different surfaces can be the right choice for improving strength and balance:

- **A forest or park floor** is soft and cushions excellently. However, roots, stones, and bumps increase the risk of injury.

- **Asphalt** is suitable for fast workouts with minimal risk of spraining. However, it stresses the joints more because it has no dampening properties. So, lightweight runners with good running technique will find asphalt to be ideal.

- **Sand** trains the muscles and lifts the feet. But, overloading the calf is possible.

- **Tartan**, a weatherproof, synthetic covering found on running tracks, is resilient, but it stresses the Achilles tendon.

- **The treadmill** offers weather-independent training on a springy surface. It requires different running motor skills because the ground rolls away from under your feet.

Start Small

Are you highly motivated to start jogging *and* are new to running? Don't!

Instead, start with walking, alternating with two minutes of jogging and two minutes of walking. Add a minute to your running interval at each training session until you can run the entire distance without a break. If two minutes are too long, go slower, gradually increasing your running over time in short intervals. Also, do the interval breaks by walking to recover. After a while, you can make the sections longer and reduce the breaks.

Don't Run Too Fast

Your body must get used to the new strain of running. So, start at a pace that's moderate enough for you to easily converse. Otherwise, frustration, overwork, pain, or even injury might result quickly. Even if you get ambitious, maintain your chosen speed for the entire route. Long-term success is only possible if you gently get your body used to the new requirements.

Take Short Steps

Running is a technically demanding sport. And more than likely, as a beginner, you'll have to adjust your technique to avoid exerting too much effort. The body develops your coordination for movement with the kilometers run.

So, try to run relaxed and with little effort. Short, easy steps are more effective than long, powerful ones, as they slow you down with each step's forward momentum.

Rest Your Body

Training for your first run was successful, and you want to start running again immediately. Great! However, *don't* start the next day: Your body needs rest to adapt to the new demands of the cardiovascular system and prepare your muscles and bones for the next running load.

Plan your training, alternating running and rest days to prevent overloading.

Remember: *Listen to your body.* Avoid pain or discomfort while running. If something doesn't feel right, stop and take a break.

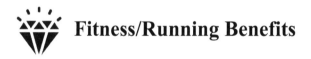 Fitness/Running Benefits

Better Blood Sugar

With regular physical exertion, you use more energy (sugar), lowering your blood sugar level and requiring less insulin. As a result, transport proteins absorb the glucose in your muscle fibers, and thus prevent diabetes mellitus. Even if you already have diabetes, you can lower your blood sugar level and possibly need less medication or insulin. Consult with your doctor before adjusting your meds.

Enhanced Sleep

Sleep better and longer with fewer disturbances when you exercise regularly for overall health.

Improved Cardiovascular Health

Sport and fitness are perfect for protecting your heart. With regular physical activity:

- Improved blood flow reduces the risk of heart disease and stroke. Endurance training, in particular, strengthens lungs and stabilizes heart muscles. This means your heart can work more economically again, and the strengthened muscles help your heart to pump more blood into your body with every beat, even receiving blood more efficiently when you take breaks.

- Blood vessels stay elastic and the risk of high blood pressure decreases. If you already have high blood pressure, you sometimes can lower it through exercise, lowering bad cholesterol (LDL) and raising good cholesterol (HDL). Consequently, you can prevent arteriosclerosis and subsequent diseases, such as stroke and heart attack.

Improved Mental Health

Exercise can reduce symptoms of anxiety and depression, and boost mood and overall well-being. And your cognitive function, including memory, attention, and decision-making abilities benefit as well.

If you participate in a sport, you'll strengthen your immune system, heart and circulation, becoming sick less often and less vulnerable to viruses and diseases. Work out a training plan to easily integrate sports into your everyday life. Remember: A fit body has tight muscles, and excess weight gradually disappears.

Increased Energy and Stamina

Exercise can boost energy levels and overall physical endurance, particularly strengthening your legs and core, as well as making daily tasks and activities easier to manage.

Increased Self-Esteem and Confidence

Your sense of accomplishment and pride in your running achievements can make you feel wonderful and powerful.

Reduced Risk of Chronic Diseases

Regular physical activity can lower the risk of chronic conditions, such as type 2 diabetes, high blood pressure, and certain types of cancer. Your strengthened immune system means you're ill less often.

Stronger Bones and Muscles

Physical activity can help improve bone density and tighten muscles, reducing the risk of osteoporosis, osteoarthritis, and falls.

Weight Management

Exercise can help burn calories, regulate weight, and reduce the risk of obesity, a culprit linked to numerous health problems.

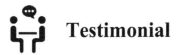 **Testimonial**

~ From author David Trofort

I reached an incredible milestone in 2021: my half-century mark. However, as a 50-year-old, I was in better shape than

20 years ago. Ironically, I can thank my unreliable, left anterior cruciate ligament (ACL). I remember it like yesterday.

It was 2010 on a Saturday night during a basketball game at our local church with pastors and elders pitted against the deacons. (Someone recruited me to participate since I served on the Music Committee.) We were warming up with basic layups when I tried to hit the backboard.

Jumping up on my left foot mid-air, bystanders heard a loud snap. Intense pain ensued and my swollen grapefruit-size knee spelled the end of my hooping days. Regrettably, I hadn't stretched before the game, and years of playing high-impact sports partly attributed to my injury. After ACL surgery, I discovered a new passion: running.

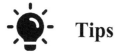 **Tips**

To get the most value from your run:

- **Set realistic goals.** Whether your goal is to run a 5K or for 30 minutes without stopping, be patient and pace yourself.

- **Stay hydrated,** drinking adequate amounts of water before, during, and after your run.

- **If you have a stitch** or pain in your side while running, breathe calmly, relax, and press your hands onto the painful area. *After* the pain subsides, run or walk slowly. Also, avoid solid food about two hours before future runs.

- **Warm up and cool down,** before and after running, with stretching exercises. Running is a workout for the whole body: "Regular strength training leads to improved running performance."

- **Mix up your sports,** such as strength training, yoga, and more, because your cardiovascular system appreciates change. In addition, the variety reduces injuries and helps you to avoid boredom.

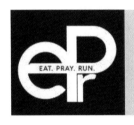

"If you can't fly, run. If you can't run, walk. If you can't walk, crawl. But by all means, keep moving."

~ Dr. Martin Luther King, Jr.

Chapter 6: Stay Motivated and Beat Obstacles

It happens to the best of us! We get excited when we embark on a new way of eating, a new or revived faith, or a different fitness routine. But because we're human, our excitement often fizzles soon afterward. Why?

Let's look at motivation, that positive or negative internal or external force that influences us to act in a certain way. For example, if we want to reach a certain income, lose 25 pounds, find enjoyment, or gain recognition, we often will act – or become motivated – to achieve that goal. And our motivation can vary – and waiver – in intensity and duration, based on our mood, mindset, values, beliefs, and environment.

Next, let's assess the motivational challenges to better prepare for conquering them:

Obstacles: Motivation Busters

Life happens. And its obstacles (be they physical, mental, emotional, or environmental) lurk around the corner, just waiting to hinder your progress. These barriers are all too familiar:

- Environmental factors, such as weather, pollution, or natural disasters

- Fear of failure

- Geographical barriers, such as mountains, rivers, or oceans, can deny access

- Limited access to specialized equipment or materials

- Limited or no financial resources

- Long distances between people and resources

- Need for more staff to assist

- Negative self-talk

- No or inadequate transportation

- Not enough time due to too many commitments

- Perfectionism (or unrealistic) expectations

- Procrastination

- Physical drawbacks, such as a chronic health issue or lack of strength

- Technological limitations, such as no or outdated hardware or software

🗪 Testimonial

~ From Ieasha A.

I've been watching and following David for quite some time, inspired by his resolve, determination, and work ethic as it relates to fitness. *Eat. Pray. Run.* is a great way to approach living your best life through faith, fitness, and food.

I've been on and off with my exercise over the past few years, but David's motivation and [social media] posts are constant reminders that real goals are attainable. He has shown that you *can* exercise, eat, and live a productive life, while taking care of yourself through running, prayer, and eating well. He doesn't judge and makes you believe in yourself. He also makes it look easy, but I know there's merited discipline through years of consistency and dedication.

Starting is the hardest part, in most cases, but he reminds me through daily encouragement.

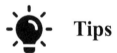 **Tips**

To stay motivated and achieve your goals:

- **Write down** specific, positively worded goals and approximate timelines to track your progress.

For example, instead of writing, "I want to lose weight," write, "I want to lose 10 pounds within two months to feel better."

- **Acknowledge** and write down which obstacle is standing in your way, such as "packed schedule," what benefit you'll gain if you achieve your goal, such as "longevity," and how you'll respond to the obstacle, such as "exercise while watching TV." Your notes will help you to build your own reference book for solutions.

- **Create or locate a workout space** that has what you need, is functional no matter the weather, and stimulates productivity.

- **Schedule your workouts** like any other appointment, incorporating taking stairs versus elevators and parking further away from buildings and storefronts.

- **Set only a few goals** or resolutions at a time to avoid frustration.

- **Expect obstacles** and setbacks from the start, asking what you can learn from the issue.

- **Divide your goal** into smaller steps to improve focus.

- **Identify, shorten, and/or eliminate time-consuming activities,** giving your goal priority.

- **Encourage yourself,** as you would your best friend, when you don't reach a goal when you'd like.

- **Practice gratitude.** There's *always* something or someone for which or for whom we can be thankful.

- **Reward yourself** appropriately for success when you reach a milestone. Doing something that brings you joy counts as self-care and generates energy for your next stage.

- **Use alternative resources,** such as online classes and partnering with like-minded, health-conscious groups, to minimize out-of-pocket costs.

- **Focus on what you *can* do,** regardless of limitations, with help from your health care provider, a professional trainer, support group, government-funded program, and/or adaptive sports, to develop a growth spirit for success.

- **Picture yourself** having reached your goals.

When things aren't going smoothly or you're feeling stuck, honestly reassess your situation and:

- **Determine whether** the original goal you set is genuinely *yours*, not someone else's.

- **Readjust your goals** to be clearer and measurable. Then change your behavior and language accordingly to hit the new target.

- **Regularly check in** with yourself via journaling or self-reflection, or seek feedback from a mentor or coach to track progress and adjust. As long as your adjustments continue to align with your overall values, vision, and long-term goals, you're okay.

- **Celebrate small wins** and defeated obstacles, whether they relate to your current goal or unrelated challenges you overcame.

- **Track data,** such as time spent, consistency, milestones, outcomes, etc., for proof of progress and to identify areas requiring more focus. Again, change how you measure progress if you need to adjust your target.

- **Discard your goal,** but only if it's unrealistic, *not* at the first sign of difficulty. This will clear the way for you to set a more practical plan with a renewed sense of purpose.

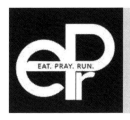

"Start where you are. Use what you have. Do what you can."

~ Arthur Ashe

Chapter 7: Love and Work

Okay, you might be as perplexed as music icon Tina Turner: "What's *love* got to do with it?" especially in a self-help book about eating, praying, and running?

Actually, love has *everything* to do with virtually *everything*, especially our health.

But don't take *my* word for it. Take *His*: "And now these three remain: faith, hope, and love. But the greatest of these is love." (1 Corinthians 13:13)

I will have been married for 17 years this November and am grateful for the love of my life, my wife Terra. She's my life partner, companion, friend, and critic. Like all couples, we've had our share of ups and downs, including balancing love and work. And as with the previous eating, praying, and running sections of this book, we must prioritize love to reap the best of what it has to offer.

Of course, no book is long enough to cover every aspect of love and work, but here's a simple plan to put and keep love at the forefront of your life:

How to Create A Love Plan

If you've ever flown before, you've heard the flight attendant instruct adults to don their own oxygen masks first, then their child's, during an emergency. In other words, you can't help someone else if you're unable to help yourself.

Here's how to apply the same, self-loving principle to the love plan you build:

- **Prioritize self-care** to maintain a healthy balance between love and work. Make time for activities that rejuvenate and recharge you.

- **Set boundaries,** ensuring that one area of life doesn't consume all of your time and energy.

- **Communicate openly and honestly with your loved ones** about your work demands and the time you need to devote to your relationship. Having a clear understanding of each other's expectations can help you find a balance that works for both of you.

- **Create a routine** that allows you to allocate time for both love and work to better manage your time and avoid feeling overwhelmed.

- **Learn to say "no"** to work-related requests that interfere with your time with loved ones. Prioritizing your relationships is just as important as your work.

- **Set realistic expectations** when work demands more of your attention than your relationship to avoid feeling guilty and prioritize your time more effectively.

- **Schedule time for your relationship** just as you schedule time for work. This will ensure that you have dedicated time to spend with your partner, while displaying that you value your relationship.

- **Delegate** some of your responsibilities to others if you have a demanding career. This will allow you to focus on your relationship and give it the time it deserves.

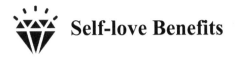 **Self-love Benefits**

Reduced Stress Levels

Self-care activities, such as meditation, yoga, or a relaxing bath can help reduce stress levels, making it easier to manage both love and work.

Improved Overall Well-being

Engaging in self-care activities can enhance our overall well-being, making it easier to manage our responsibilities.

Boosted Energy Levels

Self-care activities also can boost our energy levels, making tackling love and work easier.

Time Management Aid

Prioritizing self-care can help us manage our time better, ensuring we allocate enough time to live and work.

Increased Self-awareness

Self-care activities can let us identify our needs and better

balance life and work.

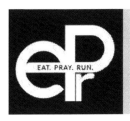

"The secret to living well and longer is to eat half, walk double, laugh triple and love without measure."

~ Tibetan Proverb

Now It's Up to You

We've explored the interconnectedness of food, faith, and fitness in this book, and their respective benefits and tips.

Remember: Incorporating healthy habits into our daily lives takes time and patience, and it's *not* about being perfect.

So, whether you're just starting your journey toward a healthier and more fulfilling life, or you're already on your way, keep moving forward, stay motivated, and never give up.

Now it's up to you! Go *Eat. Pray. Run.*

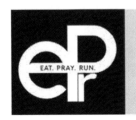

"Small changes and consistent efforts can lead to big results.

~ author David Trofort

Made in the USA
Columbia, SC
24 October 2023

24607077R00055